SATHIYA ANDIVEL

The Best Version of You

Effortless, Safe, and Natural Weight Loss for Everyone

Contents

1

Introduction

There is a moment in everyone's life when the realization hits: *I need to do something about my health.* It could be as dramatic as struggling to climb a flight of stairs or as simple as noticing your favorite jeans don't fit anymore. Perhaps it's seeing an old photo of yourself and wondering how the years managed to sneak up so fast. For some, it's a routine health check-up that delivers a wake-up call, while for others, it's the quiet realization that fatigue has become their new normal.

Whatever the trigger, the message is clear: change is needed. But here's the good news: *It's never too late—or too early—to make that change.*

A Common Misconception

One of the biggest myths about weight loss and wellness is that there's a "perfect time" to start. People in their 20s believe they'll "figure it out" in their 30s, while those in their 50s worry that it's too late to make a meaningful difference. The truth? There's no magic age when everything falls into place or when all hope is lost. The principles of health and wellness apply to everyone, at every stage of life.

Think about it: your body doesn't come with an expiration date. It's a marvel of adaptation and resilience, capable of transformation no matter how old or young you are. All it takes is the right mindset, the right approach, and a commitment to small, consistent changes.

A Universal Struggle

Let's face it: weight loss is hard. It doesn't matter if you're a college student juggling late-night study sessions or a retiree enjoying leisurely afternoons; the challenges of managing your weight are universal. Busy schedules, emotional eating, social pressures, and the sheer amount of misinformation out there can make it feel impossible to make progress.

But here's the thing: it doesn't have to be overwhelming. The journey to health doesn't require perfection, it requires consistency. And the most effective strategies aren't the ones that demand extreme sacrifices but the ones that seamlessly fit into your life.

The Goal of This Book

So, why this book? Why now? Because we're living in a time where health has become more important than ever. The world is waking up to the idea that wellness isn't just about looking good, it's about feeling good, living longer, and thriving at every stage of life.

This book is your guide to achieving exactly that. It's not about quick fixes or unsustainable crash diets. Instead, it's about equipping you with the tools, knowledge, and confidence to build a lifestyle that supports your goals—whether you're 25,

45, or 75.

Together, we'll explore:

- How your body changes with age and what that means for your weight loss journey.
- The science behind sustainable habits that actually work.
- Practical, age-inclusive strategies for nutrition, movement, and mindset.
- The importance of celebrating progress, not perfection.

And most importantly, this book is about empowerment. By the time you reach the last page, you'll not only understand how to lose weight sustainably, but you'll also feel inspired to embrace a healthier, happier version of yourself at any age.

What to Expect

In the chapters ahead, you'll find a mix of best practical experience sharing, scientific insights, and real-life examples designed to help you succeed. Whether you're just beginning your wellness journey or looking to refine your existing habits, this book offers something for everyone. Each chapter is tailored to guide you step by step, from understanding the basics of nutrition and movement to mastering the art of long-term maintenance.

Most importantly, this book is for you. It's not about one-size-fits-all solutions but about finding what works for your body, your lifestyle, and your goals.

A Shared Commitment

As you start this journey, remember: you're not alone. Thousands of people, just like you, are taking their first steps toward better health every day. What sets them apart and what will set you apart; is the willingness to start, to stay consistent, and to believe in the possibility of change.

So, here's your invitation: let's embark on this journey together. Whether you're looking to shed a few kilos, gain more energy, or simply feel more confident in your skin, know that it's possible. Your best self is waiting, and it's never too late to start.

A Note of Encouragement

As we dive into the pages ahead, let's leave behind the self-doubt, the excuses, and the guilt. Instead, let's focus on progress, growth, and the incredible potential of the human body. Every small step you take is a victory. Every healthy choice you make is a step closer to the life you deserve.

Let's begin this journey with a simple belief: *You are capable of change, and you are worth the effort.*

Welcome to the start of something amazing.

2

Why I Had to Change—and Why You Can Too

There's a moment in everyone's life when they realize things can't go on as they are. For me, that moment came during a family wedding. I was dressed in my best suits, hoping to blend into the crowd. But when the candid photos came back, I couldn't ignore what I saw. There I was, looking bloated and tired, holding a plate of sweets, fried foods, canned drinks like these were my life raft. The image haunted me; not because of how I looked but because of what it represented: years of neglecting my health, of putting everything and everyone else first, of ignoring the little signs my body had been sending me.

That photo was my wake-up call. But it wasn't the only one.

The Struggle is Real

Before I made changes, I was stuck in the same cycle so many people find themselves in. I'd try the latest crash diet, lose a few pounds, and then gain them all back, plus a little extra. I'd join a gym, go religiously for a week, and then make every excuse to skip. "I'm too busy." "I'm too tired." "I'll start again on Monday." Sound familiar?

I was constantly tired, my clothes didn't fit, and my confidence was at an all-time low. But the worst part wasn't physical—it was the mental exhaustion. I felt like I was fighting a losing battle, one where the finish line kept moving further away.

The Turning Point

That wedding photo wasn't just a reality check, it was a catalyst. It forced me to confront the truth: I wasn't just unhappy with my weight; I was unhappy with how I felt, both inside and out. I didn't have energy, I didn't feel strong, and I didn't recognize the person in the mirror. I realized I had two choices: keep making excuses or start making changes.

So, I chose change. But this time, I decided to do it differently.

The Realization That Changed Everything

Here's what I learned: weight loss isn't about suffering. It's not about starving yourself, working out until you collapse, or giving up everything you love. It's about understanding your body, making smarter choices, and building habits that actually fit your life. It's about shifting your focus from "I want to look good" to "I want to feel good."

I stopped chasing quick fixes and started focusing on what was sustainable. Instead of cutting out entire food groups, I learned how to balance my meals. Instead of punishing myself with workouts I hated, I found ways to move that felt good. And instead of aiming for perfection, I celebrated progress.

The results didn't come overnight. But they came. And they stayed.

Why This Matters to You

You might be reading this and thinking, "That's great for you, but I've tried everything, and nothing works." Trust me, I've been there. I know how frustrating it is to feel like you're spinning your wheels. But here's the thing: the problem isn't you, it's the approach you've been taught to take.

Most diets and weight loss programs are designed to fail. They rely on extremes—cutting calories too low, banning your favorite foods, or expecting you to exercise like a professional athlete. But these approaches aren't sustainable. And when they inevitably stop working, they leave you feeling like a failure.

But you're not a failure. You just need a different approach—one that's realistic, practical, and tailored to your life.

The Truth About Change

Here's what I want you to know: change is possible at any age. Your body is incredibly adaptable, no matter how many years of bad habits it's endured. You don't need perfect genetics, unlimited time, or a personal trainer to see results. What you need is the willingness to start, the patience to keep going, and the belief that you are worth the effort.

And let's clear up another myth while we're at it: weight loss isn't about deprivation. It's not about punishing yourself or giving up everything you enjoy. It's about building a life you love—one that's filled with energy, confidence, and health.

Why You Can Do This Too

If you're thinking, "I've failed so many times before; what's the point of trying again?" let me stop you right there. Every attempt you've made in the past has taught you something, even if it didn't bring you the results you wanted. And this time is different because you're not going to rely on fads or extremes. You're going to build habits that last.

This isn't about being perfect—it's about being consistent. It's about taking small, manageable steps and trusting that they will add up over time. It's about learning to listen to your body, treat it with respect, and give it what it needs to thrive.

A Journey Worth Taking

Let me be honest: this journey isn't always easy. There will be days when you feel motivated and days when you want to give up. But every step you take; no matter how small, is a victory. Every healthy choice you make is an investment in your future self.

And here's the best part: this journey isn't just about losing weight. It's about gaining so much more; energy, confidence, strength, and a deeper appreciation for what your body can do. It's about showing yourself that you are capable of change and deserving of health.

So, as you turn the page and begin this journey, I want you to hold onto one simple truth: *You can do this. You are worth it. And it's never too late to start.*

3

Who Can Join This Journey (And Who Shouldn't)

One of the most important things to understand before starting any weight loss program is this: not every approach is right for everyone. While the principles in this book are designed to be practical, sustainable, and adaptable, there are certain considerations you need to take into account. This isn't about creating limitations, it's about ensuring that the journey you embark on is safe, effective, and suited to your unique circumstances.

So, let's talk about who this program is for and who might need to take a different route or consult a professional before diving in.

Who Can Join This Journey

The beauty of this approach is that it's designed to fit into a wide range of lifestyles, ages, and situations. This program is for anyone who's ready to make small, consistent changes that lead to big results over time.

1. Healthy Adults

If you're in generally good health and looking to lose weight, improve your fitness, or simply feel better in your skin, this program is for you. Whether you're in your 20s, 40s, or 70s, the principles of sustainable weight loss; balanced nutrition, regular movement, and mindful habits are universal.

2. People Who Want a Practical Approach

This isn't a program for quick fixes or extreme sacrifices. If you're tired of fad diets that leave you feeling hungry, frustrated, and deprived, you'll find this approach refreshing. It's all about finding a rhythm that works for your life and not turning your life upside down.

3. Individuals Willing to Commit to Small Changes

Weight loss doesn't happen overnight. It requires consistency, patience, and a willingness to embrace small, incremental changes. If you're ready to focus on progress rather than perfection, you're in the right place.

4. Those Who Want to Improve Their Overall Health

This journey isn't just about shedding kilos or pounds it's about gaining energy, confidence, and a greater sense of well-being. If your goal is to feel stronger, live longer, and take control of your health, this program will guide you every step of the way.

Who Should Proceed with Caution (Or Avoid This Program)

While this approach is flexible and inclusive, there are certain groups of people for whom weight loss programs; is no matter how gentle, might not be appropriate. If you fall into any of the following categories, you may need to modify the program or seek professional guidance before starting.

1. Pregnant Women and New Mothers

Pregnancy and postpartum recovery are not the time to focus

on weight loss. Your body is going through enormous changes and needs ample nourishment to support your health and, if applicable, breastfeeding. Instead of restricting calories, focus on eating a balanced diet rich in nutrients. Once your body has recovered and you feel ready, you can explore weight management with your doctor's approval.

2. Children and Teenagers

Growing bodies have unique nutritional needs. Restrictive diets during these formative years can interfere with growth, development, and even psychological well-being. Instead of focusing on weight loss, encourage children and teens to develop healthy habits, such as eating more fruits and vegetables, staying active, and limiting processed foods.

3. Individuals with Chronic Illnesses

If you have a medical condition like diabetes, thyroid disease, heart problems, or autoimmune disorders, it's essential to consult your doctor or a registered dietitian before starting any weight loss program. These conditions require tailored plans to ensure your safety and success.

4. Differently Abled Individuals

People with physical disabilities or unique health challenges may need customized exercise and nutrition plans. While many principles in this book can be adapted, it's best to work with a healthcare professional to address specific needs.

5. People Recovering from Illness or Surgery

If you're healing from a recent illness, surgery, or injury, your body's priority is recovery—not weight loss. Focus on eating nutrient-rich foods, getting enough rest, and gradually reintroducing movement as advised by your doctor.

The Importance of Professional Guidance

If you're unsure whether this program is right for you, the best thing you can do is seek professional advice. A doctor, registered dietitian, or qualified fitness trainer can help you assess your health, set realistic goals, and adapt the program to suit your needs.

Remember: health always comes first. Weight loss should never compromise your physical or mental well-being.

A Note on Mindset

No matter who you are or where you're starting from, one thing remains true: your mindset will play a significant role in your success. This program is built on the belief that everyone; regardless of age, size, or past experiences—can improve their health and wellness. The key is to focus on what you can do, not what you can't.

If you approach this journey with an open mind, a willingness to learn, and a commitment to progress, you'll be amazed at what you can achieve.

Is This Program Right for You?

Take a moment to reflect on your current situation and your goals. Are you ready to make small, manageable changes that fit into your life? Are you prepared to focus on consistency rather than perfection? Are you willing to approach this journey with patience and positivity?

If the answer is yes, then you're exactly where you need to be. Let's get started!

4

Getting Ready to Transform

Every great journey begins with preparation. Whether you're planning a vacation, launching a new project, or starting a weight loss journey, getting ready is half the battle. The same principle applies to transforming your health and wellness—it's not just about what you do but also how you prepare your mind, body, and environment for success.

This chapter is all about setting yourself up for the journey ahead. Think of it as packing your bag with the essentials you'll need to reach your destination.

1. Setting the Right Goals

The first step to any transformation is knowing what you're working toward. But here's the key: your goals need to be realistic, specific, and meaningful.

- **Be Specific**: Saying "I want to lose weight" is vague. Instead, set measurable goals like, "I want to lose 5 kilos in 3 months" or "I want to walk 3 miles a day" or "I want to do simple work outs at home or gym"

- **Keep It Realistic**: Aim for steady progress, such as losing 0.5 to 1 kilo per week. Unrealistic goals set you up for disappointment and burnout.
- **Focus on the Bigger Picture**: Weight loss is one goal, but don't forget the deeper reasons like feeling more energetic, reducing health risks, or gaining confidence. Write these reasons down as a reminder of why you're starting this journey.

Quick Tip: Break your big goal into smaller milestones. Celebrate every achievement, no matter how small.

2. Consult a Professional

Before you begin your weight loss journey, it's crucial to consult with a doctor, dietitian, or qualified health coach. Why? Because everyone's metabolism, health history, and nutritional needs are unique. What works for one person might not work for another, and certain conditions or medications can affect your ability to lose weight or follow a specific program.

Why This Step Matters

- **Identifying Hidden Health Issues**: Conditions like hypothyroidism, PCOS, or hormonal imbalances can impact weight loss. A doctor can help diagnose and address these issues.
- **Customizing Your Plan**: A dietitian or health coach can tailor advice to suit your age, health status, and goals, ensuring your plan is both safe and effective.
- **Preventing Harm**: Restrictive diets or intense exercise programs can do more harm than good if you have specific health conditions. A professional can guide you to make informed, safe choices.

When to Seek Help

- If you have chronic health issues like diabetes, high blood pressure, or heart disease.
- If you've struggled with eating disorders in the past.
- If you're pregnant, breastfeeding, or recovering from surgery or illness.

Taking the time to consult with a professional isn't just about safety—it's about setting yourself up for success.

3. Building the Right Mindset

Weight loss is as much a mental journey as it is a physical one. Before you start, it's essential to cultivate a mindset that sets you up for long-term success.

a. Progress, Not Perfection

You're not striving to be perfect. You're striving to be better than yesterday. Accept that there will be setbacks along the way—they're part of the process. What matters is how you respond.

b. Embrace Patience

Sustainable weight loss takes time. Think of it as planting a garden: you don't see results overnight, but with consistent effort, the fruits will come.

c. Stay Positive

Instead of focusing on what you can't have, focus on what you can gain: energy, strength, confidence, and better health. Remind yourself daily that you're capable of change.

Affirmation: "I am making choices that align with my health and happiness. Every small step I take brings me closer to my goals."

4. Equipping Yourself with Tools

Like any journey, having the right tools makes all the difference. Here are some essentials to help you track progress and stay motivated:

- **A Weighing Scale**: Use it to track your weight weekly, not daily, as fluctuations are normal.
- **Measuring Tape**: Measure your waist, hips, chest, and other areas monthly. Sometimes, inches shrink even when the scale doesn't move.
- **A Food Journal or App**: Logging what you eat helps you stay mindful of your choices. Apps like MyFitnessPal can make tracking easy.
- **Comfortable Shoes**: Walking is a cornerstone of this program, so invest in a good pair of shoes.

5. Planning Your Environment

Your environment can either support or sabotage your efforts. Take some time to create a space that makes healthy choices easier.

a. Clear Out Temptations

Go through your pantry and remove items that don't align with your goals—chips, sugary snacks, and processed junk food. Out of sight, out of mind!

b. Stock Up on Essentials

Fill your kitchen with healthy staples: fruits, vegetables, whole grains, lean proteins, and nuts. Having these on hand makes it easier to prepare balanced meals.

c. Create Visual Reminders

Place motivational quotes, progress charts, or even a photo of your goal outfit in visible spots. These reminders will keep you focused on your "why."

6. Planning Your Meals and Movement

Failing to plan is planning to fail. Take some time each week to map out your meals and exercise schedule.

a. Meal Prep Basics

- Choose simple, balanced meals that include protein, fiber, and healthy fats.
- Prep ingredients ahead of time, chop veggies, cook grains, and portion out snacks.
- Keep healthy grab-and-go options, like boiled eggs, nuts, and fruit, for busy days.

b. Movement Goals

- Start with what you can manage. If 10 minutes of walking is all you can do, that's a great start.
- Build movement into your routine: take the stairs, stretch during TV commercials, or go for a walk after meals.

7. Building Your Support System

Transformation is easier when you're not doing it alone. Surround yourself with people who support your goals and encourage your efforts.

- **Share Your Goals**: Let close friends and family know about your journey. Ask for their understanding if you're making changes, like skipping late-night snacks or drinking water

instead of soda.
- **Find Accountability**: Partner with someone on a similar journey or join an online community where you can share progress and tips.

8. Preparing for Challenges

Challenges are inevitable, but planning ahead can help you navigate them with confidence.

a. Cravings and Emotional Eating

- Have healthy snacks available to combat sudden cravings.
- Distract yourself with a walk, a hobby, or a quick journaling session.

b. Social Events

- Eat a small, healthy meal beforehand so you're less tempted to overindulge.
- Focus on conversation and connection instead of food.

c. Busy Days

- Keep a stash of healthy, portable snacks like nuts, fruit, or protein bars in your bag or car.
- Remember, even 10 minutes of movement is better than none.

9. Visualizing Your Success

Finally, take a moment to picture yourself at your goal. What does your healthiest, happiest self-look like? How do you feel? What activities can you enjoy that seemed difficult before?

Hold onto this vision as your guiding light. Whenever you feel unmotivated, return to this image and remind yourself why you started.

Wrapping Up

Preparation isn't just about logistics—it's about creating a mindset and environment that make success inevitable. By taking the time to consult with professionals, set your goals, equip yourself with the right tools, and plan for challenges, you're building a foundation for transformation that lasts.

As you move forward, remember this: you don't have to be perfect. You just have to be prepared. Small, consistent efforts will take you further than you ever imagined.

Now, with your foundation set, let's dive into the habits that will drive your transformation.

Remember: I didn't begin with all these arrangements from day one. Looking back, I realize my results might have been even better if I had. Over time, as I started seeing progress, I gradually introduced these practices, one by one. So, don't feel pressured to implement everything all at once. Remember, even the smallest steps you take today are the foundation for your success tomorrow.

5

Healthy Habits: Building the Foundation for Success

The secret to lasting weight loss isn't a magic pill or an extreme diet—it's habits. Habits are the small, consistent actions that shape our daily lives. They're the reason some people seem effortlessly healthy while others struggle with every meal and every step. The good news is that habits can be built, and with time, they become second nature.

This chapter is all about laying the foundation for success by cultivating healthy habits that align with your weight loss and wellness goals. These habits aren't complicated, and they don't require drastic changes. Instead, they're practical, manageable, and designed to fit seamlessly into your life.

1. Start with Small, Achievable Changes

The biggest mistake people make when trying to lose weight is doing too much too fast. They overhaul their diet, commit to intense workouts, and set sky-high expectations—all at once. This approach often leads to burnout and frustration.

Instead, focus on small, sustainable changes. These are the

building blocks of long-term success.

Examples of Small Changes

- Drinking an extra glass of water each day.
- Adding one serving of vegetables to your meals.
- Taking a 10-minute walk after dinner.
- Swapping sugary snacks for a piece of fruit.

These changes may seem minor, but over time, they create a ripple effect that transforms your entire lifestyle.

2. Hydrate, Hydrate, Hydrate

Water is the unsung hero of weight loss. It supports digestion, helps regulate your appetite, and keeps your metabolism running smoothly. Yet, many people don't drink nearly enough.

How to Build a Hydration Habit

- Start your day with a glass of water.
- Keep a reusable water bottle with you at all times.
- Set reminders on your phone to drink a glass of water every two hours. Water could also be green tea without sugar , black coffee without sugar, butter milk, green tea but it should not be packed and preservatives added drinks
- Flavor your water with lemon, cucumber, or mint if plain water feels boring.

Aim for at least 2-3 liters of water per day, adjusting based on your activity level and climate.

3. Prioritize Protein and Fiber

When it comes to nutrition, two things should be front and

center: protein and fiber. These nutrients are the foundation of a healthy diet and play a crucial role in weight loss.

Why Protein Matters

- It keeps you full and reduces cravings.
- It helps preserve muscle mass while losing fat.
- It has a high thermic effect, meaning your body burns more calories digesting it.

Why Fiber Matters

- It slows digestion, keeping you full longer.
- It stabilizes blood sugar levels.
- It supports gut health, which is essential for overall well-being.

Simple Ways to Add Protein and Fiber to Your Diet

- Include eggs, lentils, tofu, or lean meats in your meals.
- Add chia seeds or flaxseeds to your smoothies.
- Snack on fresh fruits, nuts, or roasted chickpeas.
- Swap white rice for whole grains like red rice, quinoa or millets.

4. Make Movement a Daily Habit

Exercise doesn't have to mean gruelling gym sessions. The key is to find ways to move your body that you enjoy and to do it consistently.

Ideas for Daily Movement

- Walk for 30-40 minutes each day.
- Take the stairs instead of the elevator.
- Dance to your favorite songs for a quick mood boost.
- Try yoga or stretching to improve flexibility and reduce stress.

If you're short on time, remember that even 10-minute bursts of activity add up. The goal is to make movement a natural part of your routine.

5. Eat Mindfully

Mindful eating is the practice of paying attention to your food—what you're eating, why you're eating, and how it makes you feel. It's a simple but powerful habit that can transform your relationship with food.

How to Eat Mindfully

- Sit at a table and avoid distractions like TV or phones.
- Chew your food slowly and savor each bite.
- Stop eating when you're 80% full.
- Reflect on your hunger and fullness cues before reaching for seconds.

Mindful eating isn't about restriction—it's about awareness. The more in tune you are with your body's needs, the easier it becomes to make healthier choices.

6. Stick to Regular Meal Times

Your body thrives on routine, and sticking to consistent meal times can help regulate your metabolism and prevent overeating. Aim to eat three balanced meals a day, with snacks if needed, and finish your last meal by 6:30 PM.

Why Early Dinners Matter

- They give your body time to digest before bed.
- They help regulate hormones like insulin, which play a role in fat storage.
- They align with your body's natural circadian rhythm for better metabolism.

Plan your meals ahead of time to avoid skipping meals or resorting to unhealthy options.

7. Sleep: The Overlooked Habit

Sleep is often the missing piece in the weight loss puzzle. Poor sleep disrupts hunger hormones, increases cravings, and reduces energy for physical activity.

How to Build a Better Sleep Routine

- Go to bed and wake up at the same time every day.
- Limit screen time an hour before bed—blue light can disrupt your sleep cycle.
- Create a calming bedtime routine, like reading or meditating.
- Aim for 7-8 hours of sleep each night.

When you're well-rested, it's easier to make healthier choices and stay consistent with your habits.

8. Plan for Flexibility

Life happens. There will be days when you miss a workout, eat an unplanned snack, or feel less motivated. That's okay. The goal isn't to be perfect—it's to be consistent.

How to Stay on Track

- Have a backup plan for busy days, like a quick home workout or a healthy frozen meal.
- Don't dwell on slip-ups. Learn from them and move on.
- Focus on progress, not perfection. Even small efforts add up over time.

9. Celebrate Your Wins

Every habit you build and every milestone you reach is a step toward your goal. Take the time to celebrate your progress, whether it's losing a kilo, walking every day for a week, or simply feeling more energetic.

Non-Food Rewards

- Treat yourself to a new outfit or fitness gear.
- Plan a relaxing day off or a fun outing.
- Share your success with a friend or support group.

Celebrating your wins keeps you motivated and reminds you why you started.

10. Build Habits That Fit Your Life

Ultimately, the habits you build need to work for *you*. What fits into your schedule, your preferences, and your lifestyle? There's no one-size-fits-all approach, and that's okay. The key is to experiment, adjust, and find what feels sustainable.

Wrapping Up

Healthy habits are the foundation of success. They're the small, consistent actions that lead to big, lasting changes. By focusing on hydration, nutrition, movement, mindfulness, and sleep, you're creating a lifestyle that supports your goals—not just for today but for the years to come.

As you work on building these habits, remember: transformation doesn't happen overnight. But every healthy choice you make brings you closer to the person you want to be. Stay consistent, stay patient, and trust the process. You've got this.

6

Calories Uncovered: Eating Smart Without Guilt

Calories: they've become one of the most debated topics in the world of weight loss. Some diets tell you to count every single one, while others claim you should ignore them entirely. So, where's the truth? Somewhere in between.

Understanding calories is like understanding money in your budget. They're not inherently bad or good—they're simply units of energy. How you manage them determines whether you lose, gain, or maintain your weight. The goal of this chapter is to demystify calories and show you how to make smart, guilt-free decisions about food.

What Are Calories, Really?

A calorie is a unit of energy. Your body uses calories to fuel everything you do—breathing, walking, thinking, even sleeping. Every food and drink you consume contains calories, and your body needs a certain amount to function properly.

The Calorie Equation

- **Calories In**: The energy you consume through food and drinks.
- **Calories Out**: The energy your body burns through daily activities, exercise, and basic functions like digestion and breathing.

If you consume more calories than you burn, you store the excess as fat. If you burn more than you consume, your body uses stored fat for energy, resulting in weight loss. This is called a **calorie deficit**.

Why Counting Every Calorie Isn't Necessary

Calorie tracking can be a useful tool, especially at the beginning of your journey. But obsessing over every bite can lead to frustration and burnout. Instead of micromanaging every meal, focus on building balanced plates and being mindful of portion sizes.

The Key Is Awareness

You don't need to count every calorie to understand where they're coming from. For example:

- A handful of almonds has around 150 calories and is packed with nutrients.
- A small packet of chips has roughly the same calories but offers little nutritional value.

The goal is to choose foods that provide the most "bang for your buck"—foods that are nutrient-dense and keep you full.

Understanding Your Calorie Needs

Your calorie needs depend on several factors, including your age, gender, weight, height, and activity level. Tools like calorie calculators or consultations with a dietitian can help you estimate your daily requirements.

For sustainable weight loss, aim for a modest calorie deficit—typically 300 to 500 calories less than what your body needs to maintain its current weight. Extreme deficits may lead to rapid weight loss initially but are difficult to maintain and can harm your metabolism.

Calories Aren't the Enemy

It's important to shift your mindset about calories. They're not something to fear or avoid. Instead, think of them as fuel. The key is to choose high-quality calories that nourish your body and keep you satisfied.

Good vs. Empty Calories

- **Good Calories**: Found in nutrient-dense foods like fruits, vegetables, whole grains, lean proteins, and healthy fats. These foods provide essential vitamins, minerals, and energy.
- **Empty Calories**: Found in sugary drinks, fried foods, and processed snacks. These foods are high in calories but low in nutrients.

Choosing good calories most of the time ensures that you're fueling your body effectively while staying within your calorie budget.

Making Smart Food Choices

High-Quality Foods to Focus On

- **Protein**: Eggs, chicken, tofu, lentils, fish, Greek yogurt.
- **Fiber**: Whole grains, fruits, vegetables, legumes, nuts, seeds.
- **Healthy Fats**: Avocados, olive oil, nuts, seeds, fatty fish.
- **Hydrating Foods**: Water-rich foods like cucumbers, melons, oranges, and leafy greens.

Foods to Limit

- Sugary drinks (soda, sweetened juices).
- Deep-fried snacks (samosas, chips).
- Highly processed foods (instant noodles, packaged baked goods).

The 80/20 Rule

No one eats perfectly all the time, and you shouldn't expect to. That's where the 80/20 rule comes in:

- **80% of the time**: Focus on whole, nutrient-dense foods that align with your goals.
- **20% of the time**: Enjoy your favorite treats in moderation.

This approach helps you stay consistent without feeling deprived. Craving a slice of cake or a plate of biryani? Go for it—just make it part of your 20%.

Portion Control: The Hidden Key to Success

You can eat the healthiest foods in the world, but if you're eating double or triple the portions your body needs, you'll struggle to lose weight. Portion control doesn't mean tiny servings—it means eating the right amount for your body and goals.

Tips for Managing Portions

1. **Use Smaller Plates**: This makes servings appear larger and helps prevent overeating.
2. **Measure When Needed**: Use measuring cups or a food scale to get a sense of appropriate portions.
3. **Fill Half Your Plate with Vegetables**: They're low in calories but high in volume, helping you feel full.
4. **Practice the 80% Rule**: Stop eating when you're about 80% full.

Hidden Calories: Watch Out!

Some foods and drinks seem harmless but can secretly pack in a lot of calories. Being mindful of these can make a big difference.

Common Culprits

- Salad dressings and sauces (opt for lighter options or smaller amounts).
- Sugary coffee drinks (stick to black coffee or use minimal sugar).
- Alcoholic beverages (a single cocktail can have over 200 calories).
- Snacks labeled "healthy" (granola bars and trail mixes can be calorie-dense).

Eating Out Without Guilt

Dining out doesn't have to derail your progress. With a few smart choices, you can enjoy meals out while staying on track.

Tips for Eating Out

- **Choose Wisely**: Opt for grilled, baked, or steamed dishes instead of fried.
- **Watch Portions**: Many restaurant servings are oversized—share a dish or take leftovers home.
- **Skip the Empty Add-Ons**: Bread baskets, sugary drinks, and heavy desserts add up quickly.

Tracking Calories Without Stress

If you're new to calorie awareness, tracking your meals for a few weeks can be a helpful exercise. Apps like MyFitnessPal or Cronometer can give you insights into your eating patterns and help you make adjustments.

How to Track Without Obsessing

- Focus on trends, not daily fluctuations.
- Use tracking as a learning tool, not a rulebook.
- Stop tracking once you feel confident in your ability to make smart choices.

Guilt-Free Eating: A Mindset Shift

One of the most important lessons you'll learn is that food isn't your enemy. Eating is a natural and necessary part of life—it's how you fuel your body and connect with others. Instead of labeling foods as "good" or "bad," focus on balance.

How to Let Go of Guilt

- Practice mindful eating: Enjoy your food fully, without distractions or judgment.
- Remember the 80/20 rule: Occasional indulgences are part of a healthy lifestyle.
- Celebrate progress: Every healthy choice you make is a win, no matter how small.

Wrapping Up

Understanding calories isn't about restriction—it's about empowerment. By choosing high-quality calories, practicing portion control, and allowing room for flexibility, you can eat smart without guilt. This approach not only supports your weight loss goals but also helps you build a healthier relationship with food.

Remember: food is fuel, but it's also meant to be enjoyed. Make choices that nourish your body, satisfy your taste buds, and align with your goals. That's the essence of eating smart.

Next, we'll dive deeper into the power of food: what to embrace, what to avoid, and how to create meals that leave you feeling amazing.

7

The Power of Food: What to Embrace and What to Avoid

ood isn't just fuel—it's medicine, comfort, celebration, and culture. The choices we make at the table influence not only our weight but also our energy levels, mood, and overall health. When you embrace the right foods and limit those that don't serve your body, you set yourself up for success, one meal at a time.

This chapter is all about understanding the power of food— what to include, what to minimize, and how to strike a balance that works for you. By the end of this chapter, you'll have a clear roadmap for making food choices that align with your goals without feeling deprived.

1. The Foundation: High-Quality Foods to Embrace

Think of these foods as the building blocks of your diet. They're nutrient-dense, satisfying, and designed to fuel your body in the best possible way.

a. Protein-Rich Foods

Protein is the cornerstone of a healthy diet, especially when it comes to weight loss. It keeps you full, supports muscle maintenance, and even boosts your metabolism slightly.

- **Examples**: Eggs, chicken, turkey, fish, tofu, lentils, chickpeas, Greek yogurt, paneer, and nuts.
- **Why They Work**: Protein has a high thermic effect, meaning your body burns more calories digesting it than it does with carbs or fats.

Pro Tip: Include a source of protein in every meal to keep hunger at bay and support your weight loss efforts.

b. Fiber-Packed Foods

Fiber is your best friend for weight loss and overall health. It aids digestion, keeps you full longer, and stabilizes blood sugar levels.

- **Examples**: Whole grains (millets, quinoa, oats), fruits (berries, apples, pears), vegetables (broccoli, spinach, carrots), and legumes (black beans, kidney beans).
- **Why They Work**: Fiber slows digestion, giving you steady energy and preventing the dreaded mid-day slump.

Pro Tip: Fill half your plate with vegetables at every meal to effortlessly boost your fiber intake.

c. Healthy Fats

Not all fats are created equal. Healthy fats are essential for brain function, hormone regulation, and keeping you satisfied after meals.

- **Examples**: Avocados, olive oil, nuts, seeds, fatty fish (salmon, mackerel), and coconut oil (in moderation).
- **Why They Work**: Fats provide long-lasting energy and help your body absorb fat-soluble vitamins like A, D, E, and K.

Pro Tip: Stick to portion sizes; fats are calorie-dense, so a little goes a long way.

d. Hydrating Foods

Hydration is key to maintaining energy levels and supporting weight loss. While water is the best hydrator, many foods also contribute to your daily fluid intake.

- **Examples**: Cucumbers, watermelon, oranges, leafy greens, tomatoes.
- **Why They Work**: These foods are low in calories, high in water content, and refreshing, especially during warm weather.

e. Whole Grains

Refined grains are stripped of nutrients, but whole grains provide fiber, vitamins, and slow-releasing energy.

- **Examples**: Millets, red rice, quinoa, oats, barley.
- **Why They Work**: Whole grains stabilize blood sugar levels, preventing spikes and crashes that lead to cravings.

Pro Tip: Limit rice to once a week, and when you do eat it, choose red rice or brown rice for added nutrients.

2. Foods to Enjoy Sparingly

While no food is "forbidden," some are better enjoyed in moderation. These foods are often calorie-dense and nutrient-poor, meaning they add energy but little else to your diet.

a. Refined Carbs

These are the "quick fixes" of the food world. They give you a short burst of energy but leave you hungry soon after.

- **Examples**: White bread, white rice, sugary cereals, pastries.
- **Why Limit Them**: Refined carbs are quickly digested, causing blood sugar spikes and crashes.

b. Sugary Snacks and Beverages

Sugar is sneaky—it's hidden in more foods and drinks than you'd expect. While it's okay to indulge occasionally, frequent sugar consumption can sabotage your weight loss efforts.

- **Examples**: Soft drinks, sweetened teas, desserts, candy bars.
- **Why Limit Them**: They're high in calories and low in nutrients, often leading to weight gain and energy crashes.

c. Fried Foods

Deep-fried foods are a calorie bomb, often packed with unhealthy trans fats.

- **Examples**: Samosas, pakoras, chips, fried chicken.
- **Why Limit Them**: They're calorie-dense, hard to digest, and offer little nutritional value.

d. Processed Foods

Convenient but problematic, processed foods are often loaded with preservatives, unhealthy fats, and excess salt.

- **Examples**: Instant noodles, packaged snacks, frozen dinners.
- **Why Limit Them**: They're low in nutrients and can contribute to bloating, cravings, and weight gain.

e. Alcohol

Alcoholic drinks might seem harmless, but they're packed with empty calories and can disrupt your metabolism.

- **Examples**: Beer, wine, spirits like whisky, vodka, brandy.
- **Why Limit Them**: Alcohol slows fat burning, increases appetite, and adds unnecessary calories to your diet. Strongly recommended to avoid alcohol for at least six months till your "New You"

3. Meal Planning: Building Balanced Plates

Now that you know what to eat (and what to limit), let's talk about creating meals that are satisfying, nutrient-rich, and aligned with your goals.

Breakfast Ideas

- **Vegetable Omelet**: Packed with protein and fiber. Add spinach, tomatoes, and onions for a burst of flavor.
- **Oats with Nuts and Fruits**: A great mix of fiber, protein, and natural sweetness.

- **Boiled Eggs with Whole-Grain Toast**: A quick, filling option.

Lunch Ideas

- **Millet Roti with Vegetable Curry**: A high-fiber, nutrient-dense alternative to traditional chapati.
- **Lentil Soup with Steamed Veggies**: A protein-packed, comforting choice.
- **Salad with Paneer or Tofu**: Add olive oil and lemon dressing for flavor.

Dinner Ideas

- **Tomato Soup with Grilled Vegetables**: A light, satisfying meal.
- **Steamed Broccoli with Grilled Paneer**: High in protein and fiber.
- **Clear Vegetable Soup with a Handful of Nuts**: Great for keeping hunger at bay without overloading on calories.

4. Snacks: What to Reach For

Snacking isn't the enemy—as long as you choose wisely. Healthy snacks can prevent overeating at meals and keep your energy stable throughout the day.

- **Healthy Options**:
- A handful of nuts (almonds, walnuts).

- Fresh fruit (apple slices with peanut butter, a banana).
- Roasted chickpeas or seeds.
- **Snacks to Avoid**:
- Packaged chips.
- Sugary biscuits.
- Fried snacks like namkeen.

5. The Role of Balance

The goal isn't to eat perfectly—it's to eat better. Allow yourself to enjoy your favorite indulgences occasionally, but focus on balance. By filling your diet with nutrient-dense foods, you create room for treats without derailing your progress.

6. Tips for Success

- **Plan Ahead**: Prep meals and snacks in advance to avoid relying on unhealthy convenience foods.
- **Listen to Your Body**: Eat when you're hungry, and stop when you're satisfied—not stuffed.
- **Hydrate First**: Thirst is often mistaken for hunger. Drink water before reaching for a snack.

Wrapping Up

Food is one of the most powerful tools you have on your weight loss journey. By embracing high-quality, nutrient-dense foods and limiting processed, calorie-dense options, you create a diet that nourishes your body and fuels your goals.

Remember: this isn't about restriction—it's about choice. Choose foods that make you feel strong, energetic, and satisfied.

And when you do indulge, savor every bite without guilt. Balance is the key to a sustainable, enjoyable approach to eating.

Next, we'll dive into actionable strategies to supercharge your metabolism and help your body burn fat more efficiently.

8

The Fat-Burning Blueprint

Burning fat isn't about starving yourself or spending endless hours in the gym. It's about creating the right conditions for your body to naturally and efficiently use stored fat as fuel. Your body is designed to burn fat when you give it the right signals through nutrition, movement, and lifestyle habits.

This chapter lays out a practical, sustainable fat-burning blueprint that fits into your daily life. Think of it as a roadmap—not for quick fixes but for long-term success.

1. Understanding Fat Burning: How It Works

Fat burning happens when your body uses stored fat as energy. This process is triggered when:

- **You're in a calorie deficit**: You consume fewer calories than your body burns.
- **Insulin levels are low**: High insulin (caused by frequent snacking or sugary foods) inhibits fat burning.
- **Your metabolism is active**: An efficient metabolism helps

your body burn fat even when you're at rest.

The goal of this blueprint is to optimize these conditions.

2. Prioritize Protein at Every Meal

Protein is your best ally for fat burning. It not only helps preserve lean muscle but also increases your metabolic rate due to its high thermic effect (your body burns more calories digesting protein than carbs or fats).

How to Add More Protein

- Include eggs, lentils, tofu, paneer, or lean meats in every meal.
- Snack on Greek yogurt, nuts, or boiled eggs.
- Add protein-rich seeds like chia or flax to smoothies or salads.

3. Master Meal Timing

When you eat matters almost as much as what you eat. Aligning your meals with your body's natural rhythms can enhance fat burning.

Key Strategies

- **Finish Dinner by 6:30 PM**: This gives your body enough time to digest before sleep, allowing it to shift into fat-burning mode overnight.
- **Limit Late-Night Eating**: Nighttime snacks can disrupt your metabolism and increase fat storage.
- **Space Out Your Meals**: Avoid constant grazing. Allow gaps between meals to stabilize insulin levels and encourage fat

burning.

Pro Tip: If you feel hungry after dinner, sip on herbal tea or water to curb the craving.

4. Move After Meals

A simple 10-15 minute walk after meals can significantly improve fat burning. Post-meal movement helps your body use glucose more efficiently, reducing fat storage.

Ideas for Post-Meal Movement

- Take a leisurely walk around your neighborhood.
- Do light stretching or yoga poses.
- Pace indoors if you're short on space or time.

Why It Works: Walking after meals lowers blood sugar levels and stimulates digestion, setting the stage for fat burning.

5. Incorporate Strength Training

Building muscle is one of the most effective ways to burn fat. Muscle tissue burns more calories than fat, even at rest, which means the more muscle you have, the higher your resting metabolic rate.

Beginner-Friendly Strength Exercises

- **Bodyweight Squats**: Strengthens your legs and core.
- **Push-Ups**: Works your chest, shoulders, and arms.
- **Plank Holds**: Builds core strength and stability.
- **Lunges**: Targets your lower body and improves balance.

Start with 2-3 sessions per week, gradually increasing intensity as you get stronger.

6. Add Cardio Wisely

Cardio burns calories in the moment, but too much can lead to muscle loss, which slows your metabolism. The key is balance.

Best Cardio for Fat Burning

- **Walking**: A low-impact, sustainable option for daily movement.
- **Interval Training**: Short bursts of high-intensity activity followed by rest (e.g., jogging for 30 seconds, walking for 1 minute).
- **Dancing or Cycling**: Fun ways to get your heart rate up without feeling like a chore.

Aim for 150 minutes of moderate cardio per week, spread across multiple days.

7. Optimize Your Sleep

Sleep is a critical but often overlooked factor in fat burning. Poor sleep disrupts hormones like leptin and ghrelin, which regulate hunger and fullness, and increases cortisol, a stress hormone that promotes fat storage.

Sleep Tips for Fat Burning

- Stick to a consistent sleep schedule.
- Avoid screens an hour before bed.
- Create a calming bedtime routine (e.g., reading, meditation).
- Aim for 7–8 hours of quality sleep per night.

Why It Works: Better sleep improves your body's ability to burn fat and reduces cravings for unhealthy foods.

8. Stay Hydrated

Dehydration can slow down your metabolism and make it harder for your body to burn fat efficiently. Water also helps with digestion, reduces bloating, and supports overall energy levels.

Hydration Tips

- Drink a glass of water first thing in the morning.
- Keep a water bottle with you throughout the day.
- Drink water before meals to prevent overeating.
- Add lemon or cucumber slices for flavor.

9. Fuel Your Fat Burn with Food

Certain foods naturally boost your metabolism and encourage fat burning. Incorporate these into your meals to give your body an extra edge.

Fat-Burning Foods

- **Green Tea**: Contains catechins, which enhance metabolism.
- **Spices**: Cayenne pepper, ginger, and turmeric can slightly increase calorie burn.
- **High-Fiber Foods**: Oats, beans, and vegetables keep you full and stabilize blood sugar.
- **Healthy Fats**: Avocados and nuts help regulate hormones involved in fat metabolism.

Pro Tip: Replace sugary drinks with green tea or black coffee for a metabolism boost without added calories.

10. Manage Stress Levels

Chronic stress triggers cortisol release, which can lead to fat storage, especially around the belly. Managing stress isn't just good for your mental health—it's essential for fat burning.

Simple Stress-Relief Strategies

- Practice deep breathing or meditation for 5-10 minutes a day.
- Take breaks during work to stretch or walk.
- Spend time on hobbies that relax you.
- Connect with supportive friends or family.

Why It Works: Reducing stress improves hormone balance, making it easier for your body to shed fat.

11. Consistency Over Perfection

The key to effective fat burning isn't doing everything perfectly—it's staying consistent. Small, daily actions add up over time. Missing a workout or indulging in a treat occasionally won't derail your progress. What matters is getting back on track the next day.

12. The Big Picture

Fat burning isn't about punishing your body—it's about working with it. By combining smart nutrition, movement, and lifestyle habits, you create an environment where your body naturally uses fat as fuel. This isn't just about losing weight—it's about feeling strong, energetic, and confident in your skin.

Wrapping Up

The Fat-Burning Blueprint isn't a rigid set of rules—it's a flexible, practical guide designed to fit into your life. As you implement these strategies, remember that progress takes time. Stay patient, stay consistent, and trust that every small effort is moving you closer to your goals.

Next, we'll tackle one of the biggest challenges people face on their journey: managing cravings. Get ready to outsmart your hunger gremlins without feeling deprived.

Remember: I have intentionally repeated certain topics and concepts throughout multiple chapters because they are crucial to a successful weight loss journey. My goal is to emphasize their importance and help you internalize them, ensuring they become a natural part of your mindset and approach.

9

Craving Control: Outsmart Your Hunger Gremlins

We've all been there: a sudden craving hits, and before you know it, you're elbow-deep in a bag of chips or reaching for that last slice of cake. Cravings can feel like your worst enemy on a weight loss journey, but here's the truth—they're not as powerful as they seem.

In this chapter, we'll uncover the science behind cravings, why they happen, and, most importantly, how to outsmart them. With the right strategies, you can take control of your cravings and make them a minor detour rather than a roadblock.

1. Understanding Cravings: Why Do They Happen?

Cravings are different from hunger. While hunger is your body's signal that it needs fuel, cravings are often driven by emotions, habits, or even environmental cues.

Common Triggers for Cravings

- **Stress**: Cortisol, the stress hormone, can increase appetite and cravings for sugary or high-fat foods.

- **Boredom**: Sometimes, cravings are just a way to fill an emotional void.
- **Emotional Eating**: Sadness, anxiety, or even happiness can push you toward comfort foods.
- **Environmental Cues**: The smell of freshly baked cookies or the sight of a vending machine can trigger cravings.
- **Lack of Sleep**: Poor sleep disrupts hormones that regulate hunger, making you crave unhealthy foods.
- **Nutritional Deficiencies**: A lack of certain nutrients, like protein or magnesium, can manifest as cravings for sweets or salty snacks.

2. Recognizing Real Hunger vs. Cravings

One of the first steps to managing cravings is learning to distinguish them from true hunger.

Signs of True Hunger

- Gradual onset.
- Can be satisfied with healthy, balanced foods.
- Accompanied by physical cues like a growling stomach or low energy.

Signs of a Craving

- Sudden and specific (e.g., "I need chocolate now!").
- Persistent, even if you've eaten recently.
- Tied to emotions or situations rather than physical hunger.

Pro Tip: When a craving strikes, pause and ask yourself: "Am

I truly hungry, or is this a craving?" If it's the latter, use the strategies below to manage it.

3. Pause, Breathe, and Delay

Cravings are often fleeting, lasting only 10-15 minutes. By delaying your response, you can ride out the wave without giving in.

How to Pause and Delay

- Take a few deep breaths to calm your mind.
- Drink a glass of water—thirst is often mistaken for hunger.
- Distract yourself with an activity, like a quick walk, reading, or a phone call.

Why It Works: Delaying gives your brain time to reset, and most cravings will dissipate on their own.

4. Stay Hydrated

Dehydration can amplify cravings, especially for sugary or salty snacks. Make water your first line of defense.

Tips for Staying Hydrated

- Keep a water bottle with you and sip throughout the day.
- Flavor your water with lemon, cucumber, or mint for variety.
- Drink a glass of water before meals to help manage portion sizes.

5. Build Balanced Meals

Cravings often stem from blood sugar imbalances caused by meals that are high in refined carbs or low in nutrients.

Building balanced meals helps stabilize your blood sugar and keeps cravings at bay.

What Makes a Balanced Meal?

- **Protein**: Keeps you full and stabilizes blood sugar.
- **Fiber**: Slows digestion and prevents energy crashes.
- **Healthy Fats**: Satisfies hunger and provides lasting energy.

Example Meal: Grilled chicken with quinoa, roasted vegetables, and a drizzle of olive oil.

6. Keep Healthy Snacks on Hand

When cravings strike, having healthy alternatives ready can make all the difference. These snacks satisfy your hunger without derailing your progress.

Smart Snack Ideas

- A handful of almonds or walnuts.
- Greek yogurt with a sprinkle of chia seeds.
- Sliced apple with a tablespoon of peanut butter.
- Roasted chickpeas or seeds.

Pro Tip: Pre-portion your snacks to avoid overeating.

7. Outsmart Emotional Cravings

Emotional cravings often feel like an overwhelming need for comfort foods. The trick is to address the emotion behind the craving instead of turning to food.

How to Manage Emotional Cravings

- **Identify the Emotion**: Are you stressed, bored, or sad?

Naming the feeling can help you address it.
- **Find an Alternative Comfort**: Call a friend, journal your thoughts, or engage in a hobby.
- **Practice Mindfulness**: Sit with your feelings instead of numbing them with food. Meditation or deep breathing can help.

8. Plan for Treats

Deprivation often backfires, leading to bingeing or overindulgence later. Instead of eliminating treats entirely, plan for them in a way that feels satisfying but controlled.

How to Enjoy Treats Wisely

- Use the **80/20 Rule**: Eat nutritious, whole foods 80% of the time and allow indulgences 20% of the time.
- Opt for Smaller Portions: Share a dessert or savor a single piece of dark chocolate.
- Eat Mindfully: Focus on the taste and texture, and enjoy every bite without guilt.

Pro Tip: Treats are more satisfying when they're intentional, not impulsive.

9. Brush Your Teeth After Meals

A simple but effective trick: brushing your teeth after meals signals to your brain that eating time is over. The minty taste also makes sweet or savory foods less appealing.

10. Avoid Common Craving Triggers

Some situations or habits may set off cravings. By recognizing and avoiding these triggers, you can stay in control.

Examples of Triggers

- **Skipping Meals**: Leads to extreme hunger and poor food choices.
- **Keeping Junk Food at Home**: Out of sight, out of mind.
- **Eating While Distracted**: Watching TV or scrolling your phone during meals often leads to overeating.

11. Manage Stress Proactively

Chronic stress is a major driver of cravings, especially for sugary or high-fat foods. Incorporating stress-management techniques into your routine can reduce the frequency and intensity of cravings.

Stress-Relief Strategies

- Practice yoga or meditation for 10 minutes daily.
- Spend time in nature or go for a walk.
- Engage in a creative hobby like painting, writing, or playing music.
- Try progressive muscle relaxation or deep breathing exercises.

12. Celebrate Non-Food Victories

Cravings often come from seeking reward or comfort. Instead of turning to food, find other ways to celebrate your progress or lift your spirits.

Non-Food Rewards

- Buy yourself a new book, outfit, or gadget.
- Treat yourself to a relaxing massage or spa day.
- Take a day off to do something you love.

Pro Tip: Recognizing and celebrating your wins keeps you motivated without relying on food as a reward.

Wrapping Up

Cravings don't have to control you. By understanding why they happen and implementing strategies to manage them, you can navigate them without guilt or frustration. Remember, cravings are normal—they're not a sign of weakness or failure. The key is to stay mindful, prepared, and consistent.

As you practice these strategies, cravings will become less frequent and less intense. Over time, you'll build a stronger, healthier relationship with food—and with yourself.

Next, we'll dive into practical **Do's and Don'ts** to further solidify your weight loss journey and keep you on track.

10

Tracking Your Progress Like a Pro

Success in any journey requires knowing where you started, how far you've come, and how to keep moving forward. In weight loss and wellness, tracking progress isn't just about the numbers on a scale—it's about celebrating wins, adjusting strategies, and staying motivated.

This chapter will guide you through practical, effective ways to track your progress like a pro. By the end, you'll not only know how to measure success but also how to stay inspired throughout your journey.

1. Why Tracking Matters

Tracking your progress does more than confirm that you're heading in the right direction. It provides:

- **Clarity**: You'll understand what's working and what's not.
- **Motivation**: Seeing results, no matter how small, keeps you going.
- **Accountability**: Tracking helps you stay consistent with your efforts.

Remember, progress isn't always linear. There will be ups and downs, but tracking ensures you're moving forward overall.

2. Tools to Track Your Progress

Before diving into the methods, let's talk about tools. These simple items can help you track effectively:

- **Weighing Scale**: A staple for monitoring weight changes.
- **Measuring Tape**: Great for tracking inches lost from various parts of your body.
- **Food Diary or App**: Helps you identify eating patterns and calorie intake.
- **Fitness Tracker**: Monitors steps, workouts, and overall activity.
- **Journal**: Records non-scale victories and how you're feeling throughout the journey.

Pro Tip: Use tools that feel intuitive to you. If you're not a fan of apps, stick to a handwritten journal.

3. Tracking Weight: Do It the Right Way

Weight is one of the most common metrics people track, but it's also the most misunderstood. Daily fluctuations in water retention, hormones, and digestion can make the scale unreliable if overused.

How to Weigh Yourself Like a Pro

- Weigh yourself **once a week**, not daily.
- Choose the **same day and time** each week for consistency (e.g., Monday morning before breakfast).
- Use the **same scale** and wear similar clothing—or none at

all.
- Focus on **trends**, not single readings.

Why It Works: Weekly weigh-ins give you a clearer picture of your progress while avoiding the stress of daily fluctuations.

4. Measure Inches, Not Just Pounds

Sometimes the scale doesn't move, but your body composition changes. You might lose fat and gain muscle, which can lead to inches lost even when your weight stays the same.

How to Take Measurements

- **Waist**: Measure at the narrowest point.
- **Hips**: Measure around the widest part of your hips.
- **Chest**: Measure across the fullest part of your chest.
- **Thighs**: Measure around the thickest part of each thigh.
- **Arms**: Measure around the thickest part of your upper arms.

Pro Tip: Take measurements once a month and record them in a dedicated notebook or app.

5. Non-Scale Victories (NSVs): The Unsung Heroes

Some of the most rewarding changes aren't visible on the scale. These are called **Non-Scale Victories (NSVs)**, and they're just as important to track.

Examples of NSVs

- **Energy Levels**: You feel more energetic throughout the day.
- **Clothing Fit**: Your favorite jeans feel looser.
- **Improved Stamina**: You can climb stairs or walk longer distances without fatigue.

- **Better Sleep**: You wake up refreshed and ready to tackle the day.
- **Mental Health**: You feel more confident, focused, and positive.

Why It Matters: NSVs remind you that progress isn't just about numbers—it's about living better.

6. Take Progress Photos

Visual changes often speak louder than numbers. Taking progress photos allows you to see the transformation that might not be obvious day-to-day.

How to Take Great Progress Photos

- Stand in the **same spot** with consistent lighting.
- Wear the **same clothing** (or similar-fitting clothes) in each photo.
- Take pictures from **front, side, and back** angles.
- Repeat every 4 weeks to compare changes.

Pro Tip: Don't judge your photos too harshly—use them as a tool for self-reflection and celebration.

7. Log Your Habits, Not Just Results

Progress isn't just about the outcome—it's about the process. Tracking your habits helps you stay consistent and spot patterns that might be slowing you down.

Habits to Track

- Daily water intake.
- Meals and snacks (quality, quantity, and timing).

- Physical activity (steps, workouts, yoga).
- Sleep duration and quality.
- Stress levels and how you managed them.

Why It Works: By tracking habits, you can identify what's working and make adjustments as needed.

8. Celebrate Milestones

Every bit of progress, no matter how small, deserves recognition. Celebrating milestones keeps you motivated and reinforces positive behavior.

Examples of Milestones

- Losing your first 2 kg or 5 cm from your waist.
- Walking every day for a month.
- Completing your first strength workout.

Non-Food Rewards

- Buy yourself new workout gear or a pair of jeans in your new size.
- Treat yourself to a massage or spa day.
- Take a day off to relax and recharge.

Why It Matters: Celebrations shift your focus from "how far I have to go" to "look how far I've come."

9. Stay Flexible and Adaptable

Life happens—there will be weeks when progress slows or you face unexpected challenges. Tracking helps you adapt and stay on course.

When to Adjust Your Approach

- If weight loss stalls for several weeks, reassess your calorie intake or activity level.
- If you're feeling overly fatigued, consider increasing rest days or focusing on sleep.
- If cravings spike, review your meal balance (protein and fiber might be lacking).

Pro Tip: Use tracking as a tool for learning and adjusting, not as a reason to feel discouraged.

10. Avoid the Comparison Trap

One of the biggest pitfalls in tracking progress is comparing yourself to others. Everyone's journey is unique, and progress depends on factors like age, genetics, and lifestyle.

Focus on Your Journey

- Celebrate your own wins, no matter how small.
- Avoid social media comparisons—remember, people often share their highlights, not their struggles.
- Remind yourself of your "why" and keep your goals personal.

Why It Matters: Comparing yourself to others can lead to frustration and burnout. Your only competition is the person you were yesterday.

11. Know When to Take a Break

Tracking is a helpful tool, but it's not meant to become an obsession. If you find yourself fixating on numbers or feeling anxious about progress, it's okay to step back.

Signs You Need a Break

- Feeling stressed or overwhelmed by tracking.
- Obsessing over daily fluctuations in weight or measurements.
- Losing sight of the joy in your journey.

Pro Tip: Shift your focus to intuitive eating and movement for a while, then return to tracking when you feel ready.

12. Progress Takes Time

Weight loss and wellness are long-term journeys. Progress might feel slow at times, but every small step adds up to big results over time. Remember, the goal isn't perfection—it's consistency.

Wrapping Up

Tracking your progress is about more than numbers—it's about celebrating your journey, staying accountable, and learning what works best for your body. By combining tools like weight tracking, measurements, and NSVs with a positive mindset, you'll stay motivated and on track to reach your goals.

Remember: the journey is just as important as the destination. Celebrate every step, and trust that with consistency and patience, you're creating lasting change.

Next, we'll focus on sustaining your weight loss and transitioning into a healthy, balanced lifestyle that works for the long haul.

11

The Key to Lasting Success: Maintaining Your Results

Reaching your weight loss goal is an incredible achievement, but maintaining those results is the ultimate test of success. The truth is, the habits that helped you lose weight are the same ones that will help you keep it off. This isn't about going back to "normal"—it's about creating a new normal that feels sustainable, enjoyable, and empowering.

This chapter will guide you through the strategies, mindset shifts, and habits you need to make your results last for a lifetime.

1. Embrace the Lifestyle, Not the Diet

Many people see weight loss as a temporary phase—something to endure until they hit their goal. But sustainable success comes from embracing weight management as a lifestyle, not a quick fix.

Key Mindset Shifts

- Stop thinking of healthy eating and exercise as a "project"

with an end date.
- Focus on how these habits make you feel—energetic, confident, and strong.
- Recognize that occasional indulgences are part of the process, not a failure.

Mantra: "This is a journey, not a destination."

2. Keep Building on Your Healthy Habits

The habits you developed during your weight loss journey—balanced meals, regular movement, mindful eating—are the foundation for maintaining your results. Continue refining and adapting them to fit your evolving lifestyle.

Core Habits to Maintain

- Eating a mix of protein, fiber, and healthy fats in every meal.
- Drinking plenty of water throughout the day.
- Staying physically active, whether through walking, strength training, or a sport you enjoy.
- Getting 7-8 hours of quality sleep every night.

Pro Tip: Treat these habits as non-negotiables. They're your secret to long-term success.

3. Make Peace with the Scale

While the scale can be a useful tool, it shouldn't dictate your self-worth or success. During maintenance, your weight may fluctuate slightly, and that's perfectly normal.

How to Use the Scale Wisely

- Weigh yourself weekly, not daily, to avoid unnecessary

stress.

- Focus on trends over time rather than day-to-day changes.
- Pair weight tracking with other methods, like measurements or non-scale victories.

Mindset: "The scale is just one data point—it doesn't define me."

4. Stay Physically Active

Exercise isn't just for weight loss—it's a cornerstone of a healthy life. Staying active keeps your metabolism humming, helps manage stress, and makes you feel strong and capable.

Ways to Stay Active

- **Daily Movement**: Walking, taking the stairs, or stretching throughout the day.
- **Strength Training**: Build and maintain muscle, which burns calories even at rest.
- **Fun Activities**: Dancing, cycling, hiking—anything that keeps you moving and enjoying yourself.

Pro Tip: Find activities you love so exercise never feels like a chore.

5. Master the 80/20 Rule

The 80/20 rule is your best friend in maintenance. It means eating healthy, whole foods 80% of the time while leaving room for treats or indulgences 20% of the time. This balance prevents feelings of deprivation and keeps your lifestyle sustainable.

Examples of the 80/20 Rule

- Enjoy a slice of pizza or dessert at a party, but keep your other meals balanced.
- Treat yourself to a favorite snack once in a while without guilt.

Mantra: "Indulgence is part of balance, not the opposite of it."

6. Watch for Creeping Habits

Over time, small slips in habits—like skipping workouts or eating larger portions—can add up. Staying mindful of these shifts helps you address them before they become patterns.

How to Stay Mindful

- Check in with yourself weekly: Are you sticking to your habits?
- Journal or track your meals and activity occasionally to stay accountable.
- Set small, actionable goals to keep your focus sharp.

Pro Tip: Think of maintenance as a series of small course corrections, not a rigid plan.

7. Plan for Life's Curveballs

Vacations, holidays, and stressful times are part of life, and they often disrupt routines. The key is to navigate these moments without derailing your progress.

Strategies for Staying on Track

- **Plan Ahead**: Pack healthy snacks for trips or research restaurant menus in advance.
- **Focus on Moderation**: Enjoy holiday treats without

overindulging.

- **Get Back on Track Quickly**: One indulgent meal or skipped workout won't ruin your progress—what matters is returning to your routine.

Mindset: "It's not about perfection—it's about consistency."

8. Monitor and Celebrate Your Progress

Regularly reflecting on your journey keeps you motivated and reinforces the positive changes you've made.

Ways to Monitor Progress

- Continue tracking your weight, measurements, or fitness milestones monthly.
- Reflect on how you feel—do you have more energy, confidence, or stamina?

Celebrate Non-Scale Victories

- Fitting into clothes you love.
- Being able to do activities you couldn't before, like climbing stairs easily.
- Feeling more in control of your health and choices.

Pro Tip: Celebrate milestones with non-food rewards, like a massage, new workout gear, or a fun outing.

9. Build a Support System

Surrounding yourself with supportive people makes maintaining your results much easier. Share your journey with friends, family, or online communities to stay accountable and inspired.

How to Find Support

- Join a fitness class or walking group.
- Share your goals with a friend who can keep you motivated.
- Follow inspiring and positive health-focused accounts on social media.

Pro Tip: Be the supportive friend for someone else—you might inspire them to start their own journey.

10. Focus on How You Feel, Not Just How You Look

While weight loss might have been your initial goal, maintenance is about overall well-being. Pay attention to how your habits impact your mood, energy, and quality of life.

Signs of Success

- Waking up feeling refreshed and energetic.
- Enjoying meals without guilt or anxiety.
- Feeling more confident in your abilities and choices.

Mindset: "Health isn't just about the scale—it's about living your best life."

11. Allow Yourself Flexibility

Life changes, and so do your needs. What worked for you during weight loss might need adjustments during maintenance. Stay flexible and open to experimenting with new habits or routines.

Examples of Flexibility

- Adjust your calorie intake if your activity level changes.

- Try new recipes or exercises to keep things interesting.
- Allow yourself rest days or indulgences without guilt.

Mantra: "I'm in this for the long haul—I can adapt as needed."

12. Remember Your Why

When motivation wanes, reconnecting with your "why" can reignite your drive. Why did you start this journey? What benefits have you experienced along the way?

Your Why Might Include:

- Feeling confident in your own skin.
- Having more energy to play with your kids or enjoy your hobbies.
- Reducing health risks and living a longer, healthier life.

Pro Tip: Write down your "why" and revisit it whenever you need a boost.

Wrapping Up

Maintaining your weight loss isn't about being perfect—it's about being consistent, flexible, and kind to yourself. By continuing the habits that helped you succeed, staying mindful of your choices, and celebrating your progress, you can sustain your results for life.

The key to lasting success lies in embracing this lifestyle as a joyful, empowering journey. You've already proven you can achieve your goals—now it's time to enjoy the rewards and live the healthy, vibrant life you've worked so hard for.

12

Navigating Challenges: Staying on Track When Life Gets Tough

L ife isn't always smooth sailing. Stressful days at work, family emergencies, or unexpected setbacks can hit when you least expect them, throwing your well-laid plans into disarray. It's frustrating, no doubt. But here's the truth: challenges are part of the journey, not the end of it. The real test lies in how you respond. This chapter is about finding your footing during life's storms and staying committed to your goals, no matter how tough things get.

1. Setbacks Don't Define You

Let's start with an important reminder: everyone stumbles. Setbacks aren't a sign of failure; they're proof you're trying. It's okay to feel frustrated or disappointed, but don't let those feelings convince you to give up. Instead, remind yourself that progress is rarely a straight line.

When life gets messy, take a moment to breathe and remember why you started this journey in the first place. Acknowledge the setback, but don't dwell on it. Shift your focus to what you can do next.

2. Reconnect with Your "Why"

Your motivation, the reason you committed to this journey, can act as a powerful anchor during challenging times. Maybe it's to feel healthier, be more present for your loved ones, or regain confidence. Whatever your reason, let it guide you when things feel uncertain.

Take a moment to revisit your "why." Write it down, say it out loud, or keep a reminder where you can see it every day. Let it fuel your resolve when you're tempted to throw in the towel.

3. Simplify, Don't Overhaul

When life feels overwhelming, sticking to a perfect plan can feel impossible, and that's okay. This isn't the time for perfection. It's the time for simplicity. Focus on small, manageable actions that keep you moving forward, even if they're just baby steps.

For instance:

- If you can't cook an elaborate meal, choose a quick, nutritious option like a salad or smoothie.
- If you don't have time for a full workout, try a 10-minute walk or stretch session.
- If you're feeling too tired, focus on hydration and sleep, and let your body rest.

Small, consistent efforts add up, even during the hardest days.

4. Lean on Your People

No one succeeds alone, and you don't have to either. Whether it's a friend who cheers you on, a family member who helps lighten your load, or an online community that inspires you, lean on the people who support you.

Sometimes, just sharing what you're going through can help you feel lighter. Let others know how they can help, even if it's something as simple as listening. Remember, asking for support is a sign of strength, not weakness.

5. Be Flexible, Not Rigid

Life won't always cooperate with your plans, but that doesn't mean you have to abandon them altogether. Adaptability is your superpower. If your usual routine doesn't fit your current circumstances, tweak it.

For example:

- Swap a workout class for a quick home workout.
- Replace a meal-prep session with healthier takeout.
- Break a big goal into smaller, more achievable steps.

Flexibility allows you to keep going, even when life isn't ideal.

6. Be Kind to Yourself

Let's get real for a moment: we can be our own worst critics. When things don't go as planned, it's easy to spiral into negative self-talk. But guilt and self-criticism don't solve problems; they just make you feel worse.

Instead, treat yourself with the same kindness you'd offer a friend. If a loved one stumbled, you'd encourage them to keep going, right? Do the same for yourself. Recognize that you're doing the best you can, and that's enough.

7. Plan for the Unexpected

Preparation can make a world of difference when challenges arise. Think of it as creating a "safety net" for your goals. Having a plan in place for tough times means you'll be ready to respond, not react.

Here are some ideas to prepare:

- Keep a list of quick, healthy meals for busy days.
- Bookmark short workout videos for days when you're pressed for time.
- Develop simple stress-relief habits like journaling, deep breathing, or listening to calming music.

These small preparations can help you stay grounded, no matter what life throws your way.

8. Celebrate Your Wins (Even the Small Ones)

During tough times, progress might feel slower or even invisible. But every small victory matters. Whether it's choosing a healthier meal, taking a quick walk, or simply getting through a hard day without giving up, celebrate it.

Acknowledging your wins keeps your momentum alive and reminds you of how far you've come. Progress isn't about perfection; it's about persistence.

Final Thoughts: The Strength in Struggles

Here's the thing about challenges: they don't just test your resolve; they strengthen it. Each time you navigate a tough situation and keep moving forward, you're proving to yourself just how resilient you are.

When life gets tough, it's not about sticking to the perfect plan. It's about showing up for yourself, no matter how messy or imperfect the effort might be. Remember, your journey isn't just about the destination; it's about growing stronger and wiser along the way.

You've got this. Tough times may slow you down, but they can't stop you. Keep moving forward, one step at a time. Every step count, and every step is worth it.

Next, we'll conclude with a final chapter celebrating the new you and the endless possibilities that lie ahead.

13

Celebrating the New You

Reaching the end of a journey is always a moment worth celebrating. But in truth, the journey to a healthier, happier you; doesn't really end—it evolves. The "New You" isn't just about a number on a scale or the inches you've lost; it's about the confidence, energy, and empowerment you've gained along the way.

This chapter is a celebration of everything you've accomplished and a reminder of all the possibilities that lie ahead. Let's reflect on your transformation, honor your hard work, and inspire you to embrace the incredible life you've built.

1. Look How Far You've Come

Take a moment to pause and reflect. Think about where you started—the doubts, the struggles, the excuses that once held you back. And now, look at you. You've made changes, big and small, that have transformed not only your body but also your mindset and your life.

Signs of Your Success

- You feel stronger and more capable in your body.
- You've built habits that support your health, not sabotage it.
- You've overcome challenges and learned to adapt.
- You've inspired those around you, whether you realize it or not.

Pro Tip: Write yourself a letter about your journey—your struggles, victories, and how far you've come. Reading it in the future will remind you of your resilience and growth.

2. Celebrate Your Wins

Every milestone deserves recognition, no matter how big or small. Celebrate the inches lost, the energy gained, and the healthier choices you've made.

Creative Ways to Celebrate

- **Invest in Yourself**: Buy a new outfit that makes you feel amazing, take a class to learn something new, or indulge in a spa day.
- **Mark the Moment**: Take a progress photo, journal your thoughts, or plan a small celebration with loved ones.
- **Reward Yourself with Experiences**: Go on a hike, sign up for a fun fitness class, or treat yourself to a relaxing weekend getaway.

Why It Matters: Celebrating reinforces your success and keeps you motivated for the next phase of your journey.

3. Reflect on Your Transformation

Your physical transformation is just the beginning. The "New

You" is also about the internal changes—the resilience, self-discipline, and self-love you've cultivated.

Questions to Reflect On

- How has your confidence grown since you started?
- What challenges have you overcome, and how did you do it?
- How has your relationship with food, exercise, and your body changed?
- What are you most proud of about this journey?

Pro Tip: Share your reflections with someone who supported you along the way. It can deepen your connection and inspire them to start their own journey.

4. The Ripple Effect of Your Journey

Your transformation isn't just about you—it impacts the people around you. Whether it's your family, friends, or coworkers, your journey can inspire others to take control of their health.

Ways You've Inspired Others

- Leading by example, showing that sustainable weight loss is possible.
- Sharing tips, recipes, or workout ideas with those who ask.
- Offering support and encouragement to someone starting their own journey.

Mantra: "My journey is mine, but its impact extends far beyond me."

5. Embrace the Future with Confidence

The "New You" is just the beginning of an exciting chapter.

You've laid the foundation for a healthier life, and now it's time to build on it.
Looking Forward

- **Set New Goals**: Whether it's running a 5K, mastering a new yoga pose, or simply maintaining your results, having goals keeps you motivated.
- **Try New Things**: Experiment with recipes, activities, or hobbies that align with your lifestyle.
- **Stay Open to Growth**: Your journey will evolve as your life does. Be flexible and curious about what works best for you.

Why It Matters: Growth isn't about reaching a finish line—it's about exploring new horizons.

6. A Note on Imperfection

The "New You" isn't perfect—and that's okay. Life will throw curveballs, and there will be days when you skip a workout or indulge in a favorite treat. What matters is how you respond.
Mindset for the Future

- View slip-ups as learning experiences, not failures.
- Focus on consistency, not perfection.
- Remember that health is a journey, not a destination.

Mantra: "I'm a work in progress, and progress is beautiful."

7. Gratitude for the Journey

As you celebrate your transformation, take a moment to appreciate everything and everyone that supported your success.
Gratitude Practices

- **Thank Your Body**: It's carried you through every step of this journey.
- **Acknowledge Your Effort**: You showed up for yourself, even on hard days.
- **Appreciate Your Support System**: Whether it's friends, family, or a coach, acknowledge the people who encouraged you.

Pro Tip: Write down three things you're grateful for about your journey. Gratitude fosters a positive mindset and helps you stay motivated.

8. Parting Words of Motivation

The "New You" isn't just someone who looks different—it's someone who feels empowered to live fully. You've proven that change is possible, that you're capable of achieving your goals, and that you deserve to feel amazing in your own skin.

Final Motivation

- Keep moving forward, even when it feels hard.
- Trust the habits you've built—they're your foundation for lasting success.
- Celebrate not just who you've become, but the journey that got you here.

Wrapping Up

Congratulations on reaching this incredible milestone. You've transformed not just your body but your mindset and lifestyle. The "New You" is a testament to your hard work, dedication, and resilience.

As you move forward, remember that this isn't the end of your journey—it's the beginning of a vibrant, empowered life. Keep celebrating your wins, embracing your growth, and inspiring those around you. The best is yet to come.

Here's to the "New You" and all the amazing things you'll achieve from here on out.

14

Conclusion

As we arrive at the end of this book, it's time to pause, reflect, and look ahead. This journey to weight loss and wellness has been about so much more than the food you eat or the workouts you complete. It's about reclaiming your health, building a lifestyle that empowers you, and embracing the best version of yourself—at any age.

This chapter is not a farewell but a beginning. It's a reminder that your journey is ongoing, evolving with every step you take.

1. Reflecting on Your Transformation

Take a moment to reflect on everything you've learned and achieved. From understanding the fundamentals of weight loss to building sustainable habits, you've equipped yourself with the tools and knowledge to succeed—not just temporarily but for life.

What You've Gained

- A deeper connection with your body and its needs.
- Confidence to make informed choices about food, move-

ment, and self-care.
- A mindset focused on progress, not perfection.
- A sense of control and empowerment over your health.

Mantra: "Every step I've taken has brought me closer to the person I want to be."

2. Embracing the New You

The "New You" isn't just about the changes you see in the mirror—it's about how you feel inside. It's about the energy to chase your dreams, the confidence to stand tall, and the resilience to keep going, even when challenges arise.

Celebrating Your Wins

- Acknowledge your hard work and dedication.
- Remember the small victories, from choosing water over soda to walking instead of driving.
- Celebrate how far you've come, and let that fuel your determination to keep growing.

3. The Journey Ahead

Reaching your goals isn't the end—it's the start of a new chapter in your life. You've built a foundation of habits that will support you through life's highs and lows. As your circumstances change, so will your needs, and that's okay. Flexibility and adaptability are the keys to long-term success.

Looking Forward

- Set new goals that excite and challenge you.
- Stay curious about your body and its evolving needs.

- Share your journey with others to inspire and uplift them.

Pro Tip: Revisit this book whenever you need a reminder or a reset—it's your companion for the long haul.

4. A Final Word of Encouragement

You've proven that change is possible, that small, consistent actions can lead to extraordinary results. The most important takeaway from this journey isn't just weight loss—it's the discovery that you are capable, resilient, and deserving of a vibrant, healthy life.

Whenever doubt creeps in, remember:

- You've done hard things before—you can do them again.
- Your worth isn't defined by a number on a scale but by the joy and energy you bring to life.
- Every choice you make is a step toward becoming the best version of yourself.

5. Gratitude for the Journey

Finally, take a moment to express gratitude—for your body, which has carried you through every step of this journey; for your mind, which stayed committed even on tough days; and for the support system, whether it was friends, family, or this book, that helped you along the way.

Mantra: "I am grateful for this journey, for the lessons I've learned, and for the person I've become."

6. Parting Inspiration

Remember, you are the author of your story. This book has

been a chapter in your journey, but the pen is in your hands. Write a life filled with health, joy, and fulfillment.

"The best is yet to come."

Go forth, celebrate your success, and embrace the limitless possibilities of the "New You."

As we reach the conclusion of this transformative journey, take a moment to appreciate how far you've come—not just in terms of weight loss, but in reclaiming your health, building empowering habits, and embracing the best version of yourself. This is not just an ending; it's the dawn of new possibilities.

Reflecting on Your Transformation

You've gained more than just knowledge; you've developed a profound connection with your body, confidence in making mindful choices, and a mindset that values progress over perfection. These achievements are the foundation of your ongoing journey.

Mantra: *"Every step I've taken has brought me closer to the person I want to be."*

Embracing the New You

The changes you've made extend far beyond physical appearance. They touch every aspect of your life, giving you energy, confidence, and resilience. Celebrate every victory, big and small, and let them fuel your determination.

The Journey Ahead

The habits you've built are tools for life. As your circumstances change, so will your goals, and that's perfectly okay. Stay flexible, curious, and open to evolving alongside your needs.

Pro Tip: *This book is your companion for resets and inspiration—revisit it whenever you need guidance.*

A Final Word of Encouragement

You've proven that meaningful change is possible and that

you have the strength to overcome challenges. Remember, your worth is not tied to a number on the scale but to the vitality and joy you bring to life.

Gratitude for the Journey

Take a moment to express gratitude—to your body, which has supported you every step of the way; to your mind, which has stayed committed; and to your support system for being there when you needed it most.

Mantra: *"I am grateful for this journey, for the lessons I've learned, and for the person I've become."*

Parting Inspiration

You are the author of your story, and this book is just one chapter. The pen is in your hands to write a life filled with health, joy, and fulfillment.

Remember: *The best is yet to come.*

Thank You

Thank you for allowing this book to be part of your journey. May it continue to guide and inspire you as you embrace the limitless possibilities of the "New You."

Now, go forth and shine brightly—you've earned it.

Share Your Transformation!

Dear Reader,

Thank you for embarking on this journey with me. Your time, trust, and commitment to exploring these pages mean the world to me. I hope this book has been a valuable companion, guiding and inspiring you toward a healthier, happier, and more fulfilling life.

If this story has touched your heart, sparked a transformation, or simply provided a fresh perspective, I'd love to hear about it.

Your thoughts, feedback, and experiences not only encourage me but also help other readers discover the insights within these pages.

Here's how you can share your thoughts:

- **Leave a Review:** Write a quick review on the platform where you purchased this book. It can be as brief as a few sentences sharing what you found most impactful or why you'd recommend it to others.
- **Spread the Word:** Share your favorite takeaways on social media or with friends who might benefit from the lessons in this book. Tag me—I'd love to celebrate your journey with you!

Your review doesn't just support this book—it's a ripple that inspires others to take the first step in their transformation.

Thank you for making this journey even more meaningful. I can't wait to hear your story!

With gratitude and best wishes,
Sathiya Andivel

References:

Calorie Tracker & BMR calculator to reach your goals | MyFitness-Pal. (n.d.). https://www.myfitnesspal.com/